THIS BOOK BELONGS TO:

NAME	
ADDRESS	
PHONE #	
EMAIL	

DEDICATION

This Running Log Book is dedicated to runners who want to keep accurate records and retain information for daily runs.

You are my inspiration for producing this book and I'm honored to be a part of helping you manage and retain important information regarding your running journey.

HOW TO USE THIS BOOK

This Running Log Book will help you record, collect, and organize your information in an easy to use format.

Here are examples of information for you to fill in and write the details for your activities as a runner.

Fill in the following information:

1. Monthly Progress Pages - record weekly progress and totals, goals for the month, documents races, race and nutrition notes

2. Running Task List - record each month, use the Monday-Sunday checklist, write down tasks for each day

3. Running Log - record month, week, dates, run type, route, time, distance, pace, heart rate, calories, weather, shoes, other info, and notes

MONTHLY PROGRESS

	WEEK 1	WEEK 2	WEEK 3	WEEK 4	WEEK 5	TOTAL	AVERAGE
TOTAL MILES							
TOTAL TIME							

GOALS FOR NEXT MONTH

RACES

DATE	RACE NAME	DISTANCE	TIME	PACE	PLACE #

RACE NOTES

NUTRITION NOTES

RUNNING TASK LIST							MONTH:	
M	T	W	T	F	S	S		TASKS
								O
								O
								O
								O
								O
								O
								O
								O
								O
								O
								O
								O
								O
								O
								O
								O
								O
								O
								O
								O
								O
								O
								O
								O
								O
								O
								O
								O
								O
								O
								O

RUNNING LOG

MONTH	
WEEK #	
DATES	/ / TO / /

MONDAY

RUN TYPE						
ROUTE						
TIME		DISTANCE		PACE	
HEART RATE		CALORIES		WEATHER	
SHOES		OTHER			

TUESDAY

RUN TYPE						
ROUTE						
TIME		DISTANCE		PACE	
HEART RATE		CALORIES		WEATHER	
SHOES		OTHER			

WEDNESDAY

RUN TYPE						
ROUTE						
TIME		DISTANCE		PACE	
HEART RATE		CALORIES		WEATHER	
SHOES		OTHER			

THURSDAY

RUN TYPE						
ROUTE						
TIME		DISTANCE		PACE	
HEART RATE		CALORIES		WEATHER	
SHOES		OTHER			

RUNNING LOG

FRIDAY					
RUN TYPE					
ROUTE					
TIME		DISTANCE		PACE	
HEART RATE		CALORIES		WEATHER	
SHOES		OTHER			

SATURDAY					
RUN TYPE					
ROUTE					
TIME		DISTANCE		PACE	
HEART RATE		CALORIES		WEATHER	
SHOES		OTHER			

SUNDAY					
RUN TYPE					
ROUTE					
TIME		DISTANCE		PACE	
HEART RATE		CALORIES		WEATHER	
SHOES		OTHER			

NOTES

RUNNING LOG

MONTH	
WEEK #	
DATES	/ / TO / /

MONDAY					
RUN TYPE					
ROUTE					
TIME		DISTANCE		PACE	
HEART RATE		CALORIES		WEATHER	
SHOES		OTHER			

TUESDAY					
RUN TYPE					
ROUTE					
TIME		DISTANCE		PACE	
HEART RATE		CALORIES		WEATHER	
SHOES		OTHER			

WEDNESDAY					
RUN TYPE					
ROUTE					
TIME		DISTANCE		PACE	
HEART RATE		CALORIES		WEATHER	
SHOES		OTHER			

THURSDAY					
RUN TYPE					
ROUTE					
TIME		DISTANCE		PACE	
HEART RATE		CALORIES		WEATHER	
SHOES		OTHER			

RUNNING LOG

FRIDAY					
RUN TYPE					
ROUTE					
TIME		DISTANCE		PACE	
HEART RATE		CALORIES		WEATHER	
SHOES		OTHER			

SATURDAY					
RUN TYPE					
ROUTE					
TIME		DISTANCE		PACE	
HEART RATE		CALORIES		WEATHER	
SHOES		OTHER			

SUNDAY					
RUN TYPE					
ROUTE					
TIME		DISTANCE		PACE	
HEART RATE		CALORIES		WEATHER	
SHOES		OTHER			

NOTES

RUNNING LOG

MONTH	
WEEK #	
DATES	/ / TO / /

MONDAY					
RUN TYPE					
ROUTE					
TIME		DISTANCE		PACE	
HEART RATE		CALORIES		WEATHER	
SHOES		OTHER			

TUESDAY					
RUN TYPE					
ROUTE					
TIME		DISTANCE		PACE	
HEART RATE		CALORIES		WEATHER	
SHOES		OTHER			

WEDNESDAY					
RUN TYPE					
ROUTE					
TIME		DISTANCE		PACE	
HEART RATE		CALORIES		WEATHER	
SHOES		OTHER			

THURSDAY					
RUN TYPE					
ROUTE					
TIME		DISTANCE		PACE	
HEART RATE		CALORIES		WEATHER	
SHOES		OTHER			

RUNNING LOG

FRIDAY					
RUN TYPE					
ROUTE					
TIME		DISTANCE		PACE	
HEART RATE		CALORIES		WEATHER	
SHOES		OTHER			

SATURDAY					
RUN TYPE					
ROUTE					
TIME		DISTANCE		PACE	
HEART RATE		CALORIES		WEATHER	
SHOES		OTHER			

SUNDAY					
RUN TYPE					
ROUTE					
TIME		DISTANCE		PACE	
HEART RATE		CALORIES		WEATHER	
SHOES		OTHER			

NOTES

RUNNING LOG

MONTH	
WEEK #	
DATES	/ / TO / /

MONDAY

RUN TYPE					
ROUTE					
TIME		DISTANCE		PACE	
HEART RATE		CALORIES		WEATHER	
SHOES		OTHER			

TUESDAY

RUN TYPE					
ROUTE					
TIME		DISTANCE		PACE	
HEART RATE		CALORIES		WEATHER	
SHOES		OTHER			

WEDNESDAY

RUN TYPE					
ROUTE					
TIME		DISTANCE		PACE	
HEART RATE		CALORIES		WEATHER	
SHOES		OTHER			

THURSDAY

RUN TYPE					
ROUTE					
TIME		DISTANCE		PACE	
HEART RATE		CALORIES		WEATHER	
SHOES		OTHER			

RUNNING LOG

FRIDAY

RUN TYPE					
ROUTE					
TIME		DISTANCE		PACE	
HEART RATE		CALORIES		WEATHER	
SHOES		OTHER			

SATURDAY

RUN TYPE					
ROUTE					
TIME		DISTANCE		PACE	
HEART RATE		CALORIES		WEATHER	
SHOES		OTHER			

SUNDAY

RUN TYPE					
ROUTE					
TIME		DISTANCE		PACE	
HEART RATE		CALORIES		WEATHER	
SHOES		OTHER			

NOTES

RUNNING LOG

MONTH	
WEEK #	
DATES	/ / TO / /

MONDAY

RUN TYPE					
ROUTE					
TIME		DISTANCE		PACE	
HEART RATE		CALORIES		WEATHER	
SHOES		OTHER			

TUESDAY

RUN TYPE					
ROUTE					
TIME		DISTANCE		PACE	
HEART RATE		CALORIES		WEATHER	
SHOES		OTHER			

WEDNESDAY

RUN TYPE					
ROUTE					
TIME		DISTANCE		PACE	
HEART RATE		CALORIES		WEATHER	
SHOES		OTHER			

THURSDAY

RUN TYPE					
ROUTE					
TIME		DISTANCE		PACE	
HEART RATE		CALORIES		WEATHER	
SHOES		OTHER			

RUNNING LOG

FRIDAY

RUN TYPE					
ROUTE					
TIME		DISTANCE		PACE	
HEART RATE		CALORIES		WEATHER	
SHOES		OTHER			

SATURDAY

RUN TYPE					
ROUTE					
TIME		DISTANCE		PACE	
HEART RATE		CALORIES		WEATHER	
SHOES		OTHER			

SUNDAY

RUN TYPE					
ROUTE					
TIME		DISTANCE		PACE	
HEART RATE		CALORIES		WEATHER	
SHOES		OTHER			

NOTES

MONTHLY PROGRESS

	WEEK 1	WEEK 2	WEEK 3	WEEK 4	WEEK 5	TOTAL	AVERAGE
TOTAL MILES							
TOTAL TIME							

GOALS FOR NEXT MONTH

RACES

DATE	RACE NAME	DISTANCE	TIME	PACE	PLACE #

RACE NOTES

NUTRITION NOTES

RUNNING TASK LIST							MONTH:	
M	T	W	T	F	S	S		TASKS
							O	
							O	
							O	
							O	
							O	
							O	
							O	
							O	
							O	
							O	
							O	
							O	
							O	
							O	
							O	
							O	
							O	
							O	
							O	
							O	
							O	
							O	
							O	
							O	
							O	
							O	
							O	
							O	
							O	
							O	
							O	
							O	

RUNNING LOG

MONTH	
WEEK #	
DATES	/ / TO / /

MONDAY

RUN TYPE					
ROUTE					
TIME		DISTANCE		PACE	
HEART RATE		CALORIES		WEATHER	
SHOES		OTHER			

TUESDAY

RUN TYPE					
ROUTE					
TIME		DISTANCE		PACE	
HEART RATE		CALORIES		WEATHER	
SHOES		OTHER			

WEDNESDAY

RUN TYPE					
ROUTE					
TIME		DISTANCE		PACE	
HEART RATE		CALORIES		WEATHER	
SHOES		OTHER			

THURSDAY

RUN TYPE					
ROUTE					
TIME		DISTANCE		PACE	
HEART RATE		CALORIES		WEATHER	
SHOES		OTHER			

RUNNING LOG

FRIDAY

RUN TYPE					
ROUTE					
TIME		DISTANCE		PACE	
HEART RATE		CALORIES		WEATHER	
SHOES		OTHER			

SATURDAY

RUN TYPE					
ROUTE					
TIME		DISTANCE		PACE	
HEART RATE		CALORIES		WEATHER	
SHOES		OTHER			

SUNDAY

RUN TYPE					
ROUTE					
TIME		DISTANCE		PACE	
HEART RATE		CALORIES		WEATHER	
SHOES		OTHER			

NOTES

RUNNING LOG

MONTH	
WEEK #	
DATES	/ / TO / /

MONDAY

RUN TYPE					
ROUTE					
TIME		DISTANCE		PACE	
HEART RATE		CALORIES		WEATHER	
SHOES		OTHER			

TUESDAY

RUN TYPE					
ROUTE					
TIME		DISTANCE		PACE	
HEART RATE		CALORIES		WEATHER	
SHOES		OTHER			

WEDNESDAY

RUN TYPE					
ROUTE					
TIME		DISTANCE		PACE	
HEART RATE		CALORIES		WEATHER	
SHOES		OTHER			

THURSDAY

RUN TYPE					
ROUTE					
TIME		DISTANCE		PACE	
HEART RATE		CALORIES		WEATHER	
SHOES		OTHER			

RUNNING LOG

FRIDAY

RUN TYPE					
ROUTE					
TIME		DISTANCE		PACE	
HEART RATE		CALORIES		WEATHER	
SHOES		OTHER			

SATURDAY

RUN TYPE					
ROUTE					
TIME		DISTANCE		PACE	
HEART RATE		CALORIES		WEATHER	
SHOES		OTHER			

SUNDAY

RUN TYPE					
ROUTE					
TIME		DISTANCE		PACE	
HEART RATE		CALORIES		WEATHER	
SHOES		OTHER			

NOTES

RUNNING LOG

MONTH	
WEEK #	
DATES	/ / TO / /

MONDAY					
RUN TYPE					
ROUTE					
TIME		DISTANCE		PACE	
HEART RATE		CALORIES		WEATHER	
SHOES		OTHER			

TUESDAY					
RUN TYPE					
ROUTE					
TIME		DISTANCE		PACE	
HEART RATE		CALORIES		WEATHER	
SHOES		OTHER			

WEDNESDAY					
RUN TYPE					
ROUTE					
TIME		DISTANCE		PACE	
HEART RATE		CALORIES		WEATHER	
SHOES		OTHER			

THURSDAY					
RUN TYPE					
ROUTE					
TIME		DISTANCE		PACE	
HEART RATE		CALORIES		WEATHER	
SHOES		OTHER			

RUNNING LOG

FRIDAY					
RUN TYPE					
ROUTE					
TIME		DISTANCE		PACE	
HEART RATE		CALORIES		WEATHER	
SHOES		OTHER			

SATURDAY					
RUN TYPE					
ROUTE					
TIME		DISTANCE		PACE	
HEART RATE		CALORIES		WEATHER	
SHOES		OTHER			

SUNDAY					
RUN TYPE					
ROUTE					
TIME		DISTANCE		PACE	
HEART RATE		CALORIES		WEATHER	
SHOES		OTHER			

NOTES

RUNNING LOG

MONTH	
WEEK #	
DATES	/ / TO / /

MONDAY

RUN TYPE					
ROUTE					
TIME		DISTANCE		PACE	
HEART RATE		CALORIES		WEATHER	
SHOES		OTHER			

TUESDAY

RUN TYPE					
ROUTE					
TIME		DISTANCE		PACE	
HEART RATE		CALORIES		WEATHER	
SHOES		OTHER			

WEDNESDAY

RUN TYPE					
ROUTE					
TIME		DISTANCE		PACE	
HEART RATE		CALORIES		WEATHER	
SHOES		OTHER			

THURSDAY

RUN TYPE					
ROUTE					
TIME		DISTANCE		PACE	
HEART RATE		CALORIES		WEATHER	
SHOES		OTHER			

RUNNING LOG

FRIDAY

RUN TYPE					
ROUTE					
TIME		DISTANCE		PACE	
HEART RATE		CALORIES		WEATHER	
SHOES		OTHER			

SATURDAY

RUN TYPE					
ROUTE					
TIME		DISTANCE		PACE	
HEART RATE		CALORIES		WEATHER	
SHOES		OTHER			

SUNDAY

RUN TYPE					
ROUTE					
TIME		DISTANCE		PACE	
HEART RATE		CALORIES		WEATHER	
SHOES		OTHER			

NOTES

RUNNING LOG

MONTH	
WEEK #	
DATES	/ / TO / /

MONDAY

RUN TYPE						
ROUTE						
TIME		DISTANCE		PACE		
HEART RATE		CALORIES		WEATHER		
SHOES		OTHER				

TUESDAY

RUN TYPE						
ROUTE						
TIME		DISTANCE		PACE		
HEART RATE		CALORIES		WEATHER		
SHOES		OTHER				

WEDNESDAY

RUN TYPE						
ROUTE						
TIME		DISTANCE		PACE		
HEART RATE		CALORIES		WEATHER		
SHOES		OTHER				

THURSDAY

RUN TYPE						
ROUTE						
TIME		DISTANCE		PACE		
HEART RATE		CALORIES		WEATHER		
SHOES		OTHER				

RUNNING LOG

FRIDAY

RUN TYPE					
ROUTE					
TIME		DISTANCE		PACE	
HEART RATE		CALORIES		WEATHER	
SHOES		OTHER			

SATURDAY

RUN TYPE					
ROUTE					
TIME		DISTANCE		PACE	
HEART RATE		CALORIES		WEATHER	
SHOES		OTHER			

SUNDAY

RUN TYPE					
ROUTE					
TIME		DISTANCE		PACE	
HEART RATE		CALORIES		WEATHER	
SHOES		OTHER			

NOTES

MONTHLY PROGRESS

	WEEK 1	WEEK 2	WEEK 3	WEEK 4	WEEK 5	TOTAL	AVERAGE
TOTAL MILES							
TOTAL TIME							

GOALS FOR NEXT MONTH

RACES

DATE	RACE NAME	DISTANCE	TIME	PACE	PLACE #

RACE NOTES

NUTRITION NOTES

RUNNING TASK LIST	MONTH:						
M	T	W	T	F	S	S	TASKS
							O
							O
							O
							O
							O
							O
							O
							O
							O
							O
							O
							O
							O
							O
							O
							O
							O
							O
							O
							O
							O
							O
							O
							O
							O
							O
							O
							O
							O
							O
							O
							O
							O

RUNNING LOG

MONTH	
WEEK #	
DATES	/ / TO / /

MONDAY

RUN TYPE					
ROUTE					
TIME		DISTANCE		PACE	
HEART RATE		CALORIES		WEATHER	
SHOES		OTHER			

TUESDAY

RUN TYPE					
ROUTE					
TIME		DISTANCE		PACE	
HEART RATE		CALORIES		WEATHER	
SHOES		OTHER			

WEDNESDAY

RUN TYPE					
ROUTE					
TIME		DISTANCE		PACE	
HEART RATE		CALORIES		WEATHER	
SHOES		OTHER			

THURSDAY

RUN TYPE					
ROUTE					
TIME		DISTANCE		PACE	
HEART RATE		CALORIES		WEATHER	
SHOES		OTHER			

RUNNING LOG

FRIDAY

RUN TYPE					
ROUTE					
TIME		DISTANCE		PACE	
HEART RATE		CALORIES		WEATHER	
SHOES		OTHER			

SATURDAY

RUN TYPE					
ROUTE					
TIME		DISTANCE		PACE	
HEART RATE		CALORIES		WEATHER	
SHOES		OTHER			

SUNDAY

RUN TYPE					
ROUTE					
TIME		DISTANCE		PACE	
HEART RATE		CALORIES		WEATHER	
SHOES		OTHER			

NOTES

RUNNING LOG

MONTH	
WEEK #	
DATES	/ / TO / /

MONDAY

RUN TYPE					
ROUTE					
TIME		DISTANCE		PACE	
HEART RATE		CALORIES		WEATHER	
SHOES		OTHER			

TUESDAY

RUN TYPE					
ROUTE					
TIME		DISTANCE		PACE	
HEART RATE		CALORIES		WEATHER	
SHOES		OTHER			

WEDNESDAY

RUN TYPE					
ROUTE					
TIME		DISTANCE		PACE	
HEART RATE		CALORIES		WEATHER	
SHOES		OTHER			

THURSDAY

RUN TYPE					
ROUTE					
TIME		DISTANCE		PACE	
HEART RATE		CALORIES		WEATHER	
SHOES		OTHER			

RUNNING LOG

FRIDAY

RUN TYPE					
ROUTE					
TIME		DISTANCE		PACE	
HEART RATE		CALORIES		WEATHER	
SHOES		OTHER			

SATURDAY

RUN TYPE					
ROUTE					
TIME		DISTANCE		PACE	
HEART RATE		CALORIES		WEATHER	
SHOES		OTHER			

SUNDAY

RUN TYPE					
ROUTE					
TIME		DISTANCE		PACE	
HEART RATE		CALORIES		WEATHER	
SHOES		OTHER			

NOTES

RUNNING LOG

MONTH	
WEEK #	
DATES	/ / TO / /

MONDAY					
RUN TYPE					
ROUTE					
TIME		DISTANCE		PACE	
HEART RATE		CALORIES		WEATHER	
SHOES		OTHER			

TUESDAY					
RUN TYPE					
ROUTE					
TIME		DISTANCE		PACE	
HEART RATE		CALORIES		WEATHER	
SHOES		OTHER			

WEDNESDAY					
RUN TYPE					
ROUTE					
TIME		DISTANCE		PACE	
HEART RATE		CALORIES		WEATHER	
SHOES		OTHER			

THURSDAY					
RUN TYPE					
ROUTE					
TIME		DISTANCE		PACE	
HEART RATE		CALORIES		WEATHER	
SHOES		OTHER			

RUNNING LOG

FRIDAY

RUN TYPE					
ROUTE					
TIME		DISTANCE		PACE	
HEART RATE		CALORIES		WEATHER	
SHOES		OTHER			

SATURDAY

RUN TYPE					
ROUTE					
TIME		DISTANCE		PACE	
HEART RATE		CALORIES		WEATHER	
SHOES		OTHER			

SUNDAY

RUN TYPE					
ROUTE					
TIME		DISTANCE		PACE	
HEART RATE		CALORIES		WEATHER	
SHOES		OTHER			

NOTES

RUNNING LOG

MONTH	
WEEK #	
DATES	/ / TO / /

MONDAY

RUN TYPE						
ROUTE						
TIME		DISTANCE		PACE		
HEART RATE		CALORIES		WEATHER		
SHOES		OTHER				

TUESDAY

RUN TYPE						
ROUTE						
TIME		DISTANCE		PACE		
HEART RATE		CALORIES		WEATHER		
SHOES		OTHER				

WEDNESDAY

RUN TYPE						
ROUTE						
TIME		DISTANCE		PACE		
HEART RATE		CALORIES		WEATHER		
SHOES		OTHER				

THURSDAY

RUN TYPE						
ROUTE						
TIME		DISTANCE		PACE		
HEART RATE		CALORIES		WEATHER		
SHOES		OTHER				

RUNNING LOG

FRIDAY

RUN TYPE					
ROUTE					
TIME		DISTANCE		PACE	
HEART RATE		CALORIES		WEATHER	
SHOES		OTHER			

SATURDAY

RUN TYPE					
ROUTE					
TIME		DISTANCE		PACE	
HEART RATE		CALORIES		WEATHER	
SHOES		OTHER			

SUNDAY

RUN TYPE					
ROUTE					
TIME		DISTANCE		PACE	
HEART RATE		CALORIES		WEATHER	
SHOES		OTHER			

NOTES

RUNNING LOG

MONTH	
WEEK #	
DATES	/ / TO / /

MONDAY

RUN TYPE					
ROUTE					
TIME		DISTANCE		PACE	
HEART RATE		CALORIES		WEATHER	
SHOES		OTHER			

TUESDAY

RUN TYPE					
ROUTE					
TIME		DISTANCE		PACE	
HEART RATE		CALORIES		WEATHER	
SHOES		OTHER			

WEDNESDAY

RUN TYPE					
ROUTE					
TIME		DISTANCE		PACE	
HEART RATE		CALORIES		WEATHER	
SHOES		OTHER			

THURSDAY

RUN TYPE					
ROUTE					
TIME		DISTANCE		PACE	
HEART RATE		CALORIES		WEATHER	
SHOES		OTHER			

RUNNING LOG

FRIDAY

RUN TYPE					
ROUTE					
TIME		DISTANCE		PACE	
HEART RATE		CALORIES		WEATHER	
SHOES		OTHER			

SATURDAY

RUN TYPE					
ROUTE					
TIME		DISTANCE		PACE	
HEART RATE		CALORIES		WEATHER	
SHOES		OTHER			

SUNDAY

RUN TYPE					
ROUTE					
TIME		DISTANCE		PACE	
HEART RATE		CALORIES		WEATHER	
SHOES		OTHER			

NOTES

MONTHLY PROGRESS

	WEEK 1	WEEK 2	WEEK 3	WEEK 4	WEEK 5	TOTAL	AVERAGE
TOTAL MILES							
TOTAL TIME							

GOALS FOR NEXT MONTH

RACES

DATE	RACE NAME	DISTANCE	TIME	PACE	PLACE #

RACE NOTES

NUTRITION NOTES

RUNNING TASK LIST							MONTH:	
M	T	W	T	F	S	S		TASKS
							O	
							O	
							O	
							O	
							O	
							O	
							O	
							O	
							O	
							O	
							O	
							O	
							O	
							O	
							O	
							O	
							O	
							O	
							O	
							O	
							O	
							O	
							O	
							O	
							O	
							O	
							O	
							O	
							O	
							O	
							O	
							O	

RUNNING LOG

MONTH	
WEEK #	
DATES	/ / TO / /

MONDAY

RUN TYPE					
ROUTE					
TIME		DISTANCE		PACE	
HEART RATE		CALORIES		WEATHER	
SHOES		OTHER			

TUESDAY

RUN TYPE					
ROUTE					
TIME		DISTANCE		PACE	
HEART RATE		CALORIES		WEATHER	
SHOES		OTHER			

WEDNESDAY

RUN TYPE					
ROUTE					
TIME		DISTANCE		PACE	
HEART RATE		CALORIES		WEATHER	
SHOES		OTHER			

THURSDAY

RUN TYPE					
ROUTE					
TIME		DISTANCE		PACE	
HEART RATE		CALORIES		WEATHER	
SHOES		OTHER			

RUNNING LOG

FRIDAY

RUN TYPE					
ROUTE					
TIME		DISTANCE		PACE	
HEART RATE		CALORIES		WEATHER	
SHOES		OTHER			

SATURDAY

RUN TYPE					
ROUTE					
TIME		DISTANCE		PACE	
HEART RATE		CALORIES		WEATHER	
SHOES		OTHER			

SUNDAY

RUN TYPE					
ROUTE					
TIME		DISTANCE		PACE	
HEART RATE		CALORIES		WEATHER	
SHOES		OTHER			

NOTES

RUNNING LOG

MONTH	
WEEK #	
DATES	/ / TO / /

MONDAY

RUN TYPE					
ROUTE					
TIME		DISTANCE		PACE	
HEART RATE		CALORIES		WEATHER	
SHOES		OTHER			

TUESDAY

RUN TYPE					
ROUTE					
TIME		DISTANCE		PACE	
HEART RATE		CALORIES		WEATHER	
SHOES		OTHER			

WEDNESDAY

RUN TYPE					
ROUTE					
TIME		DISTANCE		PACE	
HEART RATE		CALORIES		WEATHER	
SHOES		OTHER			

THURSDAY

RUN TYPE					
ROUTE					
TIME		DISTANCE		PACE	
HEART RATE		CALORIES		WEATHER	
SHOES		OTHER			

RUNNING LOG

FRIDAY					
RUN TYPE					
ROUTE					
TIME		DISTANCE		PACE	
HEART RATE		CALORIES		WEATHER	
SHOES		OTHER			

SATURDAY					
RUN TYPE					
ROUTE					
TIME		DISTANCE		PACE	
HEART RATE		CALORIES		WEATHER	
SHOES		OTHER			

SUNDAY					
RUN TYPE					
ROUTE					
TIME		DISTANCE		PACE	
HEART RATE		CALORIES		WEATHER	
SHOES		OTHER			

NOTES

RUNNING LOG

MONTH	
WEEK #	
DATES	/ / TO / /

MONDAY						
RUN TYPE						
ROUTE						
TIME		DISTANCE		PACE		
HEART RATE		CALORIES		WEATHER		
SHOES		OTHER				

TUESDAY						
RUN TYPE						
ROUTE						
TIME		DISTANCE		PACE		
HEART RATE		CALORIES		WEATHER		
SHOES		OTHER				

WEDNESDAY						
RUN TYPE						
ROUTE						
TIME		DISTANCE		PACE		
HEART RATE		CALORIES		WEATHER		
SHOES		OTHER				

THURSDAY						
RUN TYPE						
ROUTE						
TIME		DISTANCE		PACE		
HEART RATE		CALORIES		WEATHER		
SHOES		OTHER				

RUNNING LOG

FRIDAY

RUN TYPE					
ROUTE					
TIME		DISTANCE		PACE	
HEART RATE		CALORIES		WEATHER	
SHOES		OTHER			

SATURDAY

RUN TYPE					
ROUTE					
TIME		DISTANCE		PACE	
HEART RATE		CALORIES		WEATHER	
SHOES		OTHER			

SUNDAY

RUN TYPE					
ROUTE					
TIME		DISTANCE		PACE	
HEART RATE		CALORIES		WEATHER	
SHOES		OTHER			

NOTES

RUNNING LOG

MONTH	
WEEK #	
DATES	/ / TO / /

MONDAY

RUN TYPE					
ROUTE					
TIME		DISTANCE		PACE	
HEART RATE		CALORIES		WEATHER	
SHOES		OTHER			

TUESDAY

RUN TYPE					
ROUTE					
TIME		DISTANCE		PACE	
HEART RATE		CALORIES		WEATHER	
SHOES		OTHER			

WEDNESDAY

RUN TYPE					
ROUTE					
TIME		DISTANCE		PACE	
HEART RATE		CALORIES		WEATHER	
SHOES		OTHER			

THURSDAY

RUN TYPE					
ROUTE					
TIME		DISTANCE		PACE	
HEART RATE		CALORIES		WEATHER	
SHOES		OTHER			

RUNNING LOG

FRIDAY					
RUN TYPE					
ROUTE					
TIME		DISTANCE		PACE	
HEART RATE		CALORIES		WEATHER	
SHOES		OTHER			

SATURDAY					
RUN TYPE					
ROUTE					
TIME		DISTANCE		PACE	
HEART RATE		CALORIES		WEATHER	
SHOES		OTHER			

SUNDAY					
RUN TYPE					
ROUTE					
TIME		DISTANCE		PACE	
HEART RATE		CALORIES		WEATHER	
SHOES		OTHER			

NOTES

RUNNING LOG

MONTH	
WEEK #	
DATES	/ / TO / /

MONDAY

RUN TYPE					
ROUTE					
TIME		DISTANCE		PACE	
HEART RATE		CALORIES		WEATHER	
SHOES		OTHER			

TUESDAY

RUN TYPE					
ROUTE					
TIME		DISTANCE		PACE	
HEART RATE		CALORIES		WEATHER	
SHOES		OTHER			

WEDNESDAY

RUN TYPE					
ROUTE					
TIME		DISTANCE		PACE	
HEART RATE		CALORIES		WEATHER	
SHOES		OTHER			

THURSDAY

RUN TYPE					
ROUTE					
TIME		DISTANCE		PACE	
HEART RATE		CALORIES		WEATHER	
SHOES		OTHER			

RUNNING LOG

FRIDAY

RUN TYPE					
ROUTE					
TIME		DISTANCE		PACE	
HEART RATE		CALORIES		WEATHER	
SHOES		OTHER			

SATURDAY

RUN TYPE					
ROUTE					
TIME		DISTANCE		PACE	
HEART RATE		CALORIES		WEATHER	
SHOES		OTHER			

SUNDAY

RUN TYPE					
ROUTE					
TIME		DISTANCE		PACE	
HEART RATE		CALORIES		WEATHER	
SHOES		OTHER			

NOTES

MONTHLY PROGRESS

	WEEK 1	WEEK 2	WEEK 3	WEEK 4	WEEK 5	TOTAL	AVERAGE
TOTAL MILES							
TOTAL TIME							

GOALS FOR NEXT MONTH

RACES					
DATE	RACE NAME	DISTANCE	TIME	PACE	PLACE #

RACE NOTES

NUTRITION NOTES

RUNNING TASK LIST	MONTH:						
M	T	W	T	F	S	S	TASKS
							O
							O
							O
							O
							O
							O
							O
							O
							O
							O
							O
							O
							O
							O
							O
							O
							O
							O
							O
							O
							O
							O
							O
							O
							O
							O
							O
							O
							O
							O
							O
							O

RUNNING LOG

MONTH	
WEEK #	
DATES	/ / TO / /

MONDAY

RUN TYPE					
ROUTE					
TIME		DISTANCE		PACE	
HEART RATE		CALORIES		WEATHER	
SHOES		OTHER			

TUESDAY

RUN TYPE					
ROUTE					
TIME		DISTANCE		PACE	
HEART RATE		CALORIES		WEATHER	
SHOES		OTHER			

WEDNESDAY

RUN TYPE					
ROUTE					
TIME		DISTANCE		PACE	
HEART RATE		CALORIES		WEATHER	
SHOES		OTHER			

THURSDAY

RUN TYPE					
ROUTE					
TIME		DISTANCE		PACE	
HEART RATE		CALORIES		WEATHER	
SHOES		OTHER			

RUNNING LOG

FRIDAY					
RUN TYPE					
ROUTE					
TIME		DISTANCE		PACE	
HEART RATE		CALORIES		WEATHER	
SHOES		OTHER			

SATURDAY					
RUN TYPE					
ROUTE					
TIME		DISTANCE		PACE	
HEART RATE		CALORIES		WEATHER	
SHOES		OTHER			

SUNDAY					
RUN TYPE					
ROUTE					
TIME		DISTANCE		PACE	
HEART RATE		CALORIES		WEATHER	
SHOES		OTHER			

NOTES

RUNNING LOG

MONTH	
WEEK #	
DATES	/ / TO / /

MONDAY

RUN TYPE					
ROUTE					
TIME		DISTANCE		PACE	
HEART RATE		CALORIES		WEATHER	
SHOES		OTHER			

TUESDAY

RUN TYPE					
ROUTE					
TIME		DISTANCE		PACE	
HEART RATE		CALORIES		WEATHER	
SHOES		OTHER			

WEDNESDAY

RUN TYPE					
ROUTE					
TIME		DISTANCE		PACE	
HEART RATE		CALORIES		WEATHER	
SHOES		OTHER			

THURSDAY

RUN TYPE					
ROUTE					
TIME		DISTANCE		PACE	
HEART RATE		CALORIES		WEATHER	
SHOES		OTHER			

RUNNING LOG

FRIDAY

RUN TYPE					
ROUTE					
TIME		DISTANCE		PACE	
HEART RATE		CALORIES		WEATHER	
SHOES		OTHER			

SATURDAY

RUN TYPE					
ROUTE					
TIME		DISTANCE		PACE	
HEART RATE		CALORIES		WEATHER	
SHOES		OTHER			

SUNDAY

RUN TYPE					
ROUTE					
TIME		DISTANCE		PACE	
HEART RATE		CALORIES		WEATHER	
SHOES		OTHER			

NOTES

RUNNING LOG

MONTH	
WEEK #	
DATES	/ / TO / /

MONDAY

RUN TYPE					
ROUTE					
TIME		DISTANCE		PACE	
HEART RATE		CALORIES		WEATHER	
SHOES		OTHER			

TUESDAY

RUN TYPE					
ROUTE					
TIME		DISTANCE		PACE	
HEART RATE		CALORIES		WEATHER	
SHOES		OTHER			

WEDNESDAY

RUN TYPE					
ROUTE					
TIME		DISTANCE		PACE	
HEART RATE		CALORIES		WEATHER	
SHOES		OTHER			

THURSDAY

RUN TYPE					
ROUTE					
TIME		DISTANCE		PACE	
HEART RATE		CALORIES		WEATHER	
SHOES		OTHER			

RUNNING LOG

FRIDAY					
RUN TYPE					
ROUTE					
TIME		DISTANCE		PACE	
HEART RATE		CALORIES		WEATHER	
SHOES		OTHER			

SATURDAY					
RUN TYPE					
ROUTE					
TIME		DISTANCE		PACE	
HEART RATE		CALORIES		WEATHER	
SHOES		OTHER			

SUNDAY					
RUN TYPE					
ROUTE					
TIME		DISTANCE		PACE	
HEART RATE		CALORIES		WEATHER	
SHOES		OTHER			

NOTES

RUNNING LOG

MONTH	
WEEK #	
DATES	/ / TO / /

MONDAY

RUN TYPE						
ROUTE						
TIME		DISTANCE		PACE	
HEART RATE		CALORIES		WEATHER	
SHOES		OTHER			

TUESDAY

RUN TYPE						
ROUTE						
TIME		DISTANCE		PACE	
HEART RATE		CALORIES		WEATHER	
SHOES		OTHER			

WEDNESDAY

RUN TYPE						
ROUTE						
TIME		DISTANCE		PACE	
HEART RATE		CALORIES		WEATHER	
SHOES		OTHER			

THURSDAY

RUN TYPE						
ROUTE						
TIME		DISTANCE		PACE	
HEART RATE		CALORIES		WEATHER	
SHOES		OTHER			

RUNNING LOG

FRIDAY					
RUN TYPE					
ROUTE					
TIME		DISTANCE		PACE	
HEART RATE		CALORIES		WEATHER	
SHOES		OTHER			

SATURDAY					
RUN TYPE					
ROUTE					
TIME		DISTANCE		PACE	
HEART RATE		CALORIES		WEATHER	
SHOES		OTHER			

SUNDAY					
RUN TYPE					
ROUTE					
TIME		DISTANCE		PACE	
HEART RATE		CALORIES		WEATHER	
SHOES		OTHER			

NOTES

RUNNING LOG

MONTH	
WEEK #	
DATES	/ / TO / /

MONDAY

RUN TYPE					
ROUTE					
TIME		DISTANCE		PACE	
HEART RATE		CALORIES		WEATHER	
SHOES		OTHER			

TUESDAY

RUN TYPE					
ROUTE					
TIME		DISTANCE		PACE	
HEART RATE		CALORIES		WEATHER	
SHOES		OTHER			

WEDNESDAY

RUN TYPE					
ROUTE					
TIME		DISTANCE		PACE	
HEART RATE		CALORIES		WEATHER	
SHOES		OTHER			

THURSDAY

RUN TYPE					
ROUTE					
TIME		DISTANCE		PACE	
HEART RATE		CALORIES		WEATHER	
SHOES		OTHER			

RUNNING LOG

FRIDAY					
RUN TYPE					
ROUTE					
TIME		DISTANCE		PACE	
HEART RATE		CALORIES		WEATHER	
SHOES		OTHER			

SATURDAY					
RUN TYPE					
ROUTE					
TIME		DISTANCE		PACE	
HEART RATE		CALORIES		WEATHER	
SHOES		OTHER			

SUNDAY					
RUN TYPE					
ROUTE					
TIME		DISTANCE		PACE	
HEART RATE		CALORIES		WEATHER	
SHOES		OTHER			

NOTES

MONTHLY PROGRESS

	WEEK 1	WEEK 2	WEEK 3	WEEK 4	WEEK 5	TOTAL	AVERAGE
TOTAL MILES							
TOTAL TIME							

GOALS FOR NEXT MONTH

RACES

DATE	RACE NAME	DISTANCE	TIME	PACE	PLACE #

RACE NOTES

NUTRITION NOTES

RUNNING TASK LIST							MONTH:	
M	T	W	T	F	S	S	TASKS	
							O	
							O	
							O	
							O	
							O	
							O	
							O	
							O	
							O	
							O	
							O	
							O	
							O	
							O	
							O	
							O	
							O	
							O	
							O	
							O	
							O	
							O	
							O	
							O	
							O	
							O	
							O	
							O	
							O	
							O	

RUNNING LOG

MONTH	
WEEK #	
DATES	/ / TO / /

MONDAY					
RUN TYPE					
ROUTE					
TIME		DISTANCE		PACE	
HEART RATE		CALORIES		WEATHER	
SHOES		OTHER			

TUESDAY					
RUN TYPE					
ROUTE					
TIME		DISTANCE		PACE	
HEART RATE		CALORIES		WEATHER	
SHOES		OTHER			

WEDNESDAY					
RUN TYPE					
ROUTE					
TIME		DISTANCE		PACE	
HEART RATE		CALORIES		WEATHER	
SHOES		OTHER			

THURSDAY					
RUN TYPE					
ROUTE					
TIME		DISTANCE		PACE	
HEART RATE		CALORIES		WEATHER	
SHOES		OTHER			

RUNNING LOG

FRIDAY					
RUN TYPE					
ROUTE					
TIME		DISTANCE		PACE	
HEART RATE		CALORIES		WEATHER	
SHOES		OTHER			

SATURDAY					
RUN TYPE					
ROUTE					
TIME		DISTANCE		PACE	
HEART RATE		CALORIES		WEATHER	
SHOES		OTHER			

SUNDAY					
RUN TYPE					
ROUTE					
TIME		DISTANCE		PACE	
HEART RATE		CALORIES		WEATHER	
SHOES		OTHER			

NOTES

RUNNING LOG

MONTH	
WEEK #	
DATES	/ / TO / /

MONDAY

RUN TYPE					
ROUTE					
TIME		DISTANCE		PACE	
HEART RATE		CALORIES		WEATHER	
SHOES		OTHER			

TUESDAY

RUN TYPE					
ROUTE					
TIME		DISTANCE		PACE	
HEART RATE		CALORIES		WEATHER	
SHOES		OTHER			

WEDNESDAY

RUN TYPE					
ROUTE					
TIME		DISTANCE		PACE	
HEART RATE		CALORIES		WEATHER	
SHOES		OTHER			

THURSDAY

RUN TYPE					
ROUTE					
TIME		DISTANCE		PACE	
HEART RATE		CALORIES		WEATHER	
SHOES		OTHER			

RUNNING LOG

FRIDAY

RUN TYPE					
ROUTE					
TIME		DISTANCE		PACE	
HEART RATE		CALORIES		WEATHER	
SHOES		OTHER			

SATURDAY

RUN TYPE					
ROUTE					
TIME		DISTANCE		PACE	
HEART RATE		CALORIES		WEATHER	
SHOES		OTHER			

SUNDAY

RUN TYPE					
ROUTE					
TIME		DISTANCE		PACE	
HEART RATE		CALORIES		WEATHER	
SHOES		OTHER			

NOTES

RUNNING LOG

MONTH	
WEEK #	
DATES	/ / TO / /

MONDAY

RUN TYPE					
ROUTE					
TIME		DISTANCE		PACE	
HEART RATE		CALORIES		WEATHER	
SHOES		OTHER			

TUESDAY

RUN TYPE					
ROUTE					
TIME		DISTANCE		PACE	
HEART RATE		CALORIES		WEATHER	
SHOES		OTHER			

WEDNESDAY

RUN TYPE					
ROUTE					
TIME		DISTANCE		PACE	
HEART RATE		CALORIES		WEATHER	
SHOES		OTHER			

THURSDAY

RUN TYPE					
ROUTE					
TIME		DISTANCE		PACE	
HEART RATE		CALORIES		WEATHER	
SHOES		OTHER			

RUNNING LOG

FRIDAY					
RUN TYPE					
ROUTE					
TIME		DISTANCE		PACE	
HEART RATE		CALORIES		WEATHER	
SHOES		OTHER			

SATURDAY					
RUN TYPE					
ROUTE					
TIME		DISTANCE		PACE	
HEART RATE		CALORIES		WEATHER	
SHOES		OTHER			

SUNDAY					
RUN TYPE					
ROUTE					
TIME		DISTANCE		PACE	
HEART RATE		CALORIES		WEATHER	
SHOES		OTHER			

NOTES

RUNNING LOG

MONTH	
WEEK #	
DATES	/ / TO / /

MONDAY

RUN TYPE					
ROUTE					
TIME		DISTANCE		PACE	
HEART RATE		CALORIES		WEATHER	
SHOES		OTHER			

TUESDAY

RUN TYPE					
ROUTE					
TIME		DISTANCE		PACE	
HEART RATE		CALORIES		WEATHER	
SHOES		OTHER			

WEDNESDAY

RUN TYPE					
ROUTE					
TIME		DISTANCE		PACE	
HEART RATE		CALORIES		WEATHER	
SHOES		OTHER			

THURSDAY

RUN TYPE					
ROUTE					
TIME		DISTANCE		PACE	
HEART RATE		CALORIES		WEATHER	
SHOES		OTHER			

RUNNING LOG

FRIDAY					
RUN TYPE					
ROUTE					
TIME		DISTANCE		PACE	
HEART RATE		CALORIES		WEATHER	
SHOES		OTHER			

SATURDAY					
RUN TYPE					
ROUTE					
TIME		DISTANCE		PACE	
HEART RATE		CALORIES		WEATHER	
SHOES		OTHER			

SUNDAY					
RUN TYPE					
ROUTE					
TIME		DISTANCE		PACE	
HEART RATE		CALORIES		WEATHER	
SHOES		OTHER			

NOTES

RUNNING LOG

MONTH	
WEEK #	
DATES	/ / TO / /

MONDAY

RUN TYPE					
ROUTE					
TIME		DISTANCE		PACE	
HEART RATE		CALORIES		WEATHER	
SHOES		OTHER			

TUESDAY

RUN TYPE					
ROUTE					
TIME		DISTANCE		PACE	
HEART RATE		CALORIES		WEATHER	
SHOES		OTHER			

WEDNESDAY

RUN TYPE					
ROUTE					
TIME		DISTANCE		PACE	
HEART RATE		CALORIES		WEATHER	
SHOES		OTHER			

THURSDAY

RUN TYPE					
ROUTE					
TIME		DISTANCE		PACE	
HEART RATE		CALORIES		WEATHER	
SHOES		OTHER			

RUNNING LOG

FRIDAY

RUN TYPE					
ROUTE					
TIME		DISTANCE		PACE	
HEART RATE		CALORIES		WEATHER	
SHOES		OTHER			

SATURDAY

RUN TYPE					
ROUTE					
TIME		DISTANCE		PACE	
HEART RATE		CALORIES		WEATHER	
SHOES		OTHER			

SUNDAY

RUN TYPE					
ROUTE					
TIME		DISTANCE		PACE	
HEART RATE		CALORIES		WEATHER	
SHOES		OTHER			

NOTES

MONTHLY PROGRESS

	WEEK 1	WEEK 2	WEEK 3	WEEK 4	WEEK 5	TOTAL	AVERAGE
TOTAL MILES							
TOTAL TIME							

GOALS FOR NEXT MONTH

RACES

DATE	RACE NAME	DISTANCE	TIME	PACE	PLACE #

RACE NOTES

NUTRITION NOTES

RUNNING TASK LIST							MONTH:
M	T	W	T	F	S	S	TASKS
							O
							O
							O
							O
							O
							O
							O
							O
							O
							O
							O
							O
							O
							O
							O
							O
							O
							O
							O
							O
							O
							O
							O
							O
							O
							O
							O
							O
							O
							O

RUNNING LOG

MONTH	
WEEK #	
DATES	/ / TO / /

MONDAY

RUN TYPE					
ROUTE					
TIME		DISTANCE		PACE	
HEART RATE		CALORIES		WEATHER	
SHOES		OTHER			

TUESDAY

RUN TYPE					
ROUTE					
TIME		DISTANCE		PACE	
HEART RATE		CALORIES		WEATHER	
SHOES		OTHER			

WEDNESDAY

RUN TYPE					
ROUTE					
TIME		DISTANCE		PACE	
HEART RATE		CALORIES		WEATHER	
SHOES		OTHER			

THURSDAY

RUN TYPE					
ROUTE					
TIME		DISTANCE		PACE	
HEART RATE		CALORIES		WEATHER	
SHOES		OTHER			

RUNNING LOG

FRIDAY

RUN TYPE					
ROUTE					
TIME		DISTANCE		PACE	
HEART RATE		CALORIES		WEATHER	
SHOES		OTHER			

SATURDAY

RUN TYPE					
ROUTE					
TIME		DISTANCE		PACE	
HEART RATE		CALORIES		WEATHER	
SHOES		OTHER			

SUNDAY

RUN TYPE					
ROUTE					
TIME		DISTANCE		PACE	
HEART RATE		CALORIES		WEATHER	
SHOES		OTHER			

NOTES

RUNNING LOG

MONTH	
WEEK #	
DATES	/ / TO / /

MONDAY

RUN TYPE					
ROUTE					
TIME		DISTANCE		PACE	
HEART RATE		CALORIES		WEATHER	
SHOES		OTHER			

TUESDAY

RUN TYPE					
ROUTE					
TIME		DISTANCE		PACE	
HEART RATE		CALORIES		WEATHER	
SHOES		OTHER			

WEDNESDAY

RUN TYPE					
ROUTE					
TIME		DISTANCE		PACE	
HEART RATE		CALORIES		WEATHER	
SHOES		OTHER			

THURSDAY

RUN TYPE					
ROUTE					
TIME		DISTANCE		PACE	
HEART RATE		CALORIES		WEATHER	
SHOES		OTHER			

RUNNING LOG

FRIDAY					
RUN TYPE					
ROUTE					
TIME		DISTANCE		PACE	
HEART RATE		CALORIES		WEATHER	
SHOES		OTHER			

SATURDAY					
RUN TYPE					
ROUTE					
TIME		DISTANCE		PACE	
HEART RATE		CALORIES		WEATHER	
SHOES		OTHER			

SUNDAY					
RUN TYPE					
ROUTE					
TIME		DISTANCE		PACE	
HEART RATE		CALORIES		WEATHER	
SHOES		OTHER			

NOTES

RUNNING LOG

MONTH	
WEEK #	
DATES	/ / TO / /

MONDAY						
RUN TYPE						
ROUTE						
TIME		DISTANCE		PACE		
HEART RATE		CALORIES		WEATHER		
SHOES		OTHER				

TUESDAY						
RUN TYPE						
ROUTE						
TIME		DISTANCE		PACE		
HEART RATE		CALORIES		WEATHER		
SHOES		OTHER				

WEDNESDAY						
RUN TYPE						
ROUTE						
TIME		DISTANCE		PACE		
HEART RATE		CALORIES		WEATHER		
SHOES		OTHER				

THURSDAY						
RUN TYPE						
ROUTE						
TIME		DISTANCE		PACE		
HEART RATE		CALORIES		WEATHER		
SHOES		OTHER				

RUNNING LOG

FRIDAY					
RUN TYPE					
ROUTE					
TIME		DISTANCE		PACE	
HEART RATE		CALORIES		WEATHER	
SHOES		OTHER			

SATURDAY					
RUN TYPE					
ROUTE					
TIME		DISTANCE		PACE	
HEART RATE		CALORIES		WEATHER	
SHOES		OTHER			

SUNDAY					
RUN TYPE					
ROUTE					
TIME		DISTANCE		PACE	
HEART RATE		CALORIES		WEATHER	
SHOES		OTHER			

NOTES

RUNNING LOG

MONTH	
WEEK #	
DATES	/ / TO / /

MONDAY

RUN TYPE					
ROUTE					
TIME		DISTANCE		PACE	
HEART RATE		CALORIES		WEATHER	
SHOES		OTHER			

TUESDAY

RUN TYPE					
ROUTE					
TIME		DISTANCE		PACE	
HEART RATE		CALORIES		WEATHER	
SHOES		OTHER			

WEDNESDAY

RUN TYPE					
ROUTE					
TIME		DISTANCE		PACE	
HEART RATE		CALORIES		WEATHER	
SHOES		OTHER			

THURSDAY

RUN TYPE					
ROUTE					
TIME		DISTANCE		PACE	
HEART RATE		CALORIES		WEATHER	
SHOES		OTHER			

RUNNING LOG

FRIDAY					
RUN TYPE					
ROUTE					
TIME		DISTANCE		PACE	
HEART RATE		CALORIES		WEATHER	
SHOES		OTHER			

SATURDAY					
RUN TYPE					
ROUTE					
TIME		DISTANCE		PACE	
HEART RATE		CALORIES		WEATHER	
SHOES		OTHER			

SUNDAY					
RUN TYPE					
ROUTE					
TIME		DISTANCE		PACE	
HEART RATE		CALORIES		WEATHER	
SHOES		OTHER			

NOTES

RUNNING LOG

MONTH	
WEEK #	
DATES	/ / TO / /

MONDAY

RUN TYPE					
ROUTE					
TIME		DISTANCE		PACE	
HEART RATE		CALORIES		WEATHER	
SHOES		OTHER			

TUESDAY

RUN TYPE					
ROUTE					
TIME		DISTANCE		PACE	
HEART RATE		CALORIES		WEATHER	
SHOES		OTHER			

WEDNESDAY

RUN TYPE					
ROUTE					
TIME		DISTANCE		PACE	
HEART RATE		CALORIES		WEATHER	
SHOES		OTHER			

THURSDAY

RUN TYPE					
ROUTE					
TIME		DISTANCE		PACE	
HEART RATE		CALORIES		WEATHER	
SHOES		OTHER			

RUNNING LOG

FRIDAY

RUN TYPE					
ROUTE					
TIME		DISTANCE		PACE	
HEART RATE		CALORIES		WEATHER	
SHOES		OTHER			

SATURDAY

RUN TYPE					
ROUTE					
TIME		DISTANCE		PACE	
HEART RATE		CALORIES		WEATHER	
SHOES		OTHER			

SUNDAY

RUN TYPE					
ROUTE					
TIME		DISTANCE		PACE	
HEART RATE		CALORIES		WEATHER	
SHOES		OTHER			

NOTES

MONTHLY PROGRESS

	WEEK 1	WEEK 2	WEEK 3	WEEK 4	WEEK 5	TOTAL	AVERAGE
TOTAL MILES							
TOTAL TIME							

GOALS FOR NEXT MONTH

RACES

DATE	RACE NAME	DISTANCE	TIME	PACE	PLACE #

RACE NOTES

NUTRITION NOTES

RUNNING TASK LIST							MONTH:
M	T	W	T	F	S	S	TASKS
							O
							O
							O
							O
							O
							O
							O
							O
							O
							O
							O
							O
							O
							O
							O
							O
							O
							O
							O
							O
							O
							O
							O
							O
							O
							O
							O
							O
							O
							O
							O
							O

RUNNING LOG

MONTH	
WEEK #	
DATES	/ / TO / /

MONDAY

RUN TYPE					
ROUTE					
TIME		DISTANCE		PACE	
HEART RATE		CALORIES		WEATHER	
SHOES		OTHER			

TUESDAY

RUN TYPE					
ROUTE					
TIME		DISTANCE		PACE	
HEART RATE		CALORIES		WEATHER	
SHOES		OTHER			

WEDNESDAY

RUN TYPE					
ROUTE					
TIME		DISTANCE		PACE	
HEART RATE		CALORIES		WEATHER	
SHOES		OTHER			

THURSDAY

RUN TYPE					
ROUTE					
TIME		DISTANCE		PACE	
HEART RATE		CALORIES		WEATHER	
SHOES		OTHER			

RUNNING LOG

FRIDAY					
RUN TYPE					
ROUTE					
TIME		DISTANCE		PACE	
HEART RATE		CALORIES		WEATHER	
SHOES		OTHER			

SATURDAY					
RUN TYPE					
ROUTE					
TIME		DISTANCE		PACE	
HEART RATE		CALORIES		WEATHER	
SHOES		OTHER			

SUNDAY					
RUN TYPE					
ROUTE					
TIME		DISTANCE		PACE	
HEART RATE		CALORIES		WEATHER	
SHOES		OTHER			

NOTES

RUNNING LOG

MONTH	
WEEK #	
DATES	/ / TO / /

MONDAY

RUN TYPE						
ROUTE						
TIME		DISTANCE		PACE		
HEART RATE		CALORIES		WEATHER		
SHOES		OTHER				

TUESDAY

RUN TYPE						
ROUTE						
TIME		DISTANCE		PACE		
HEART RATE		CALORIES		WEATHER		
SHOES		OTHER				

WEDNESDAY

RUN TYPE						
ROUTE						
TIME		DISTANCE		PACE		
HEART RATE		CALORIES		WEATHER		
SHOES		OTHER				

THURSDAY

RUN TYPE						
ROUTE						
TIME		DISTANCE		PACE		
HEART RATE		CALORIES		WEATHER		
SHOES		OTHER				

RUNNING LOG

FRIDAY

RUN TYPE					
ROUTE					
TIME		DISTANCE		PACE	
HEART RATE		CALORIES		WEATHER	
SHOES		OTHER			

SATURDAY

RUN TYPE					
ROUTE					
TIME		DISTANCE		PACE	
HEART RATE		CALORIES		WEATHER	
SHOES		OTHER			

SUNDAY

RUN TYPE					
ROUTE					
TIME		DISTANCE		PACE	
HEART RATE		CALORIES		WEATHER	
SHOES		OTHER			

NOTES

RUNNING LOG

MONTH	
WEEK #	
DATES	/ / TO / /

MONDAY

RUN TYPE						
ROUTE						
TIME		DISTANCE		PACE		
HEART RATE		CALORIES		WEATHER		
SHOES		OTHER				

TUESDAY

RUN TYPE						
ROUTE						
TIME		DISTANCE		PACE		
HEART RATE		CALORIES		WEATHER		
SHOES		OTHER				

WEDNESDAY

RUN TYPE						
ROUTE						
TIME		DISTANCE		PACE		
HEART RATE		CALORIES		WEATHER		
SHOES		OTHER				

THURSDAY

RUN TYPE						
ROUTE						
TIME		DISTANCE		PACE		
HEART RATE		CALORIES		WEATHER		
SHOES		OTHER				

RUNNING LOG

FRIDAY

RUN TYPE					
ROUTE					
TIME		DISTANCE		PACE	
HEART RATE		CALORIES		WEATHER	
SHOES		OTHER			

SATURDAY

RUN TYPE					
ROUTE					
TIME		DISTANCE		PACE	
HEART RATE		CALORIES		WEATHER	
SHOES		OTHER			

SUNDAY

RUN TYPE					
ROUTE					
TIME		DISTANCE		PACE	
HEART RATE		CALORIES		WEATHER	
SHOES		OTHER			

NOTES

RUNNING LOG

MONTH	
WEEK #	
DATES	/ / TO / /

MONDAY

RUN TYPE					
ROUTE					
TIME		DISTANCE		PACE	
HEART RATE		CALORIES		WEATHER	
SHOES		OTHER			

TUESDAY

RUN TYPE					
ROUTE					
TIME		DISTANCE		PACE	
HEART RATE		CALORIES		WEATHER	
SHOES		OTHER			

WEDNESDAY

RUN TYPE					
ROUTE					
TIME		DISTANCE		PACE	
HEART RATE		CALORIES		WEATHER	
SHOES		OTHER			

THURSDAY

RUN TYPE					
ROUTE					
TIME		DISTANCE		PACE	
HEART RATE		CALORIES		WEATHER	
SHOES		OTHER			

RUNNING LOG

FRIDAY					
RUN TYPE					
ROUTE					
TIME		DISTANCE		PACE	
HEART RATE		CALORIES		WEATHER	
SHOES		OTHER			

SATURDAY					
RUN TYPE					
ROUTE					
TIME		DISTANCE		PACE	
HEART RATE		CALORIES		WEATHER	
SHOES		OTHER			

SUNDAY					
RUN TYPE					
ROUTE					
TIME		DISTANCE		PACE	
HEART RATE		CALORIES		WEATHER	
SHOES		OTHER			

NOTES

RUNNING LOG

MONTH	
WEEK #	
DATES	/ / TO / /

MONDAY					
RUN TYPE					
ROUTE					
TIME		DISTANCE		PACE	
HEART RATE		CALORIES		WEATHER	
SHOES		OTHER			

TUESDAY					
RUN TYPE					
ROUTE					
TIME		DISTANCE		PACE	
HEART RATE		CALORIES		WEATHER	
SHOES		OTHER			

WEDNESDAY					
RUN TYPE					
ROUTE					
TIME		DISTANCE		PACE	
HEART RATE		CALORIES		WEATHER	
SHOES		OTHER			

THURSDAY					
RUN TYPE					
ROUTE					
TIME		DISTANCE		PACE	
HEART RATE		CALORIES		WEATHER	
SHOES		OTHER			

RUNNING LOG

FRIDAY					
RUN TYPE					
ROUTE					
TIME		DISTANCE		PACE	
HEART RATE		CALORIES		WEATHER	
SHOES		OTHER			

SATURDAY					
RUN TYPE					
ROUTE					
TIME		DISTANCE		PACE	
HEART RATE		CALORIES		WEATHER	
SHOES		OTHER			

SUNDAY					
RUN TYPE					
ROUTE					
TIME		DISTANCE		PACE	
HEART RATE		CALORIES		WEATHER	
SHOES		OTHER			

NOTES

MONTHLY PROGRESS

	WEEK 1	WEEK 2	WEEK 3	WEEK 4	WEEK 5	TOTAL	AVERAGE
TOTAL MILES							
TOTAL TIME							

GOALS FOR NEXT MONTH

RACES

DATE	RACE NAME	DISTANCE	TIME	PACE	PLACE #

RACE NOTES

NUTRITION NOTES

RUNNING TASK LIST							MONTH:
M	T	W	T	F	S	S	TASKS
							O
							O
							O
							O
							O
							O
							O
							O
							O
							O
							O
							O
							O
							O
							O
							O
							O
							O
							O
							O
							O
							O
							O
							O
							O
							O
							O
							O
							O
							O
							O
							O

RUNNING LOG

MONTH	
WEEK #	
DATES	/　　　/　　　TO　　　/　　　/

MONDAY

RUN TYPE						
ROUTE						
TIME		DISTANCE		PACE	
HEART RATE		CALORIES		WEATHER	
SHOES		OTHER			

TUESDAY

RUN TYPE						
ROUTE						
TIME		DISTANCE		PACE	
HEART RATE		CALORIES		WEATHER	
SHOES		OTHER			

WEDNESDAY

RUN TYPE						
ROUTE						
TIME		DISTANCE		PACE	
HEART RATE		CALORIES		WEATHER	
SHOES		OTHER			

THURSDAY

RUN TYPE						
ROUTE						
TIME		DISTANCE		PACE	
HEART RATE		CALORIES		WEATHER	
SHOES		OTHER			

RUNNING LOG

FRIDAY

RUN TYPE					
ROUTE					
TIME		DISTANCE		PACE	
HEART RATE		CALORIES		WEATHER	
SHOES		OTHER			

SATURDAY

RUN TYPE					
ROUTE					
TIME		DISTANCE		PACE	
HEART RATE		CALORIES		WEATHER	
SHOES		OTHER			

SUNDAY

RUN TYPE					
ROUTE					
TIME		DISTANCE		PACE	
HEART RATE		CALORIES		WEATHER	
SHOES		OTHER			

NOTES

RUNNING LOG

MONTH	
WEEK #	
DATES	/ / TO / /

MONDAY					
RUN TYPE					
ROUTE					
TIME		DISTANCE		PACE	
HEART RATE		CALORIES		WEATHER	
SHOES		OTHER			

TUESDAY					
RUN TYPE					
ROUTE					
TIME		DISTANCE		PACE	
HEART RATE		CALORIES		WEATHER	
SHOES		OTHER			

WEDNESDAY					
RUN TYPE					
ROUTE					
TIME		DISTANCE		PACE	
HEART RATE		CALORIES		WEATHER	
SHOES		OTHER			

THURSDAY					
RUN TYPE					
ROUTE					
TIME		DISTANCE		PACE	
HEART RATE		CALORIES		WEATHER	
SHOES		OTHER			

RUNNING LOG

FRIDAY

RUN TYPE						
ROUTE						
TIME		DISTANCE		PACE		
HEART RATE		CALORIES		WEATHER		
SHOES		OTHER				

SATURDAY

RUN TYPE						
ROUTE						
TIME		DISTANCE		PACE		
HEART RATE		CALORIES		WEATHER		
SHOES		OTHER				

SUNDAY

RUN TYPE						
ROUTE						
TIME		DISTANCE		PACE		
HEART RATE		CALORIES		WEATHER		
SHOES		OTHER				

NOTES

RUNNING LOG

MONTH	
WEEK #	
DATES	/ / TO / /

MONDAY						
RUN TYPE						
ROUTE						
TIME		DISTANCE		PACE		
HEART RATE		CALORIES		WEATHER		
SHOES		OTHER				

TUESDAY						
RUN TYPE						
ROUTE						
TIME		DISTANCE		PACE		
HEART RATE		CALORIES		WEATHER		
SHOES		OTHER				

WEDNESDAY						
RUN TYPE						
ROUTE						
TIME		DISTANCE		PACE		
HEART RATE		CALORIES		WEATHER		
SHOES		OTHER				

THURSDAY						
RUN TYPE						
ROUTE						
TIME		DISTANCE		PACE		
HEART RATE		CALORIES		WEATHER		
SHOES		OTHER				

RUNNING LOG

FRIDAY

RUN TYPE						
ROUTE						
TIME		DISTANCE		PACE		
HEART RATE		CALORIES		WEATHER		
SHOES		OTHER				

SATURDAY

RUN TYPE						
ROUTE						
TIME		DISTANCE		PACE		
HEART RATE		CALORIES		WEATHER		
SHOES		OTHER				

SUNDAY

RUN TYPE						
ROUTE						
TIME		DISTANCE		PACE		
HEART RATE		CALORIES		WEATHER		
SHOES		OTHER				

NOTES

RUNNING LOG

MONTH	
WEEK #	
DATES	/ / TO / /

MONDAY					
RUN TYPE					
ROUTE					
TIME		DISTANCE		PACE	
HEART RATE		CALORIES		WEATHER	
SHOES		OTHER			

TUESDAY					
RUN TYPE					
ROUTE					
TIME		DISTANCE		PACE	
HEART RATE		CALORIES		WEATHER	
SHOES		OTHER			

WEDNESDAY					
RUN TYPE					
ROUTE					
TIME		DISTANCE		PACE	
HEART RATE		CALORIES		WEATHER	
SHOES		OTHER			

THURSDAY					
RUN TYPE					
ROUTE					
TIME		DISTANCE		PACE	
HEART RATE		CALORIES		WEATHER	
SHOES		OTHER			

RUNNING LOG

FRIDAY

RUN TYPE					
ROUTE					
TIME		DISTANCE		PACE	
HEART RATE		CALORIES		WEATHER	
SHOES		OTHER			

SATURDAY

RUN TYPE					
ROUTE					
TIME		DISTANCE		PACE	
HEART RATE		CALORIES		WEATHER	
SHOES		OTHER			

SUNDAY

RUN TYPE					
ROUTE					
TIME		DISTANCE		PACE	
HEART RATE		CALORIES		WEATHER	
SHOES		OTHER			

NOTES

RUNNING LOG

MONTH	
WEEK #	
DATES	/ / TO / /

MONDAY					
RUN TYPE					
ROUTE					
TIME		DISTANCE		PACE	
HEART RATE		CALORIES		WEATHER	
SHOES		OTHER			

TUESDAY					
RUN TYPE					
ROUTE					
TIME		DISTANCE		PACE	
HEART RATE		CALORIES		WEATHER	
SHOES		OTHER			

WEDNESDAY					
RUN TYPE					
ROUTE					
TIME		DISTANCE		PACE	
HEART RATE		CALORIES		WEATHER	
SHOES		OTHER			

THURSDAY					
RUN TYPE					
ROUTE					
TIME		DISTANCE		PACE	
HEART RATE		CALORIES		WEATHER	
SHOES		OTHER			

RUNNING LOG

FRIDAY					
RUN TYPE					
ROUTE					
TIME		DISTANCE		PACE	
HEART RATE		CALORIES		WEATHER	
SHOES		OTHER			

SATURDAY					
RUN TYPE					
ROUTE					
TIME		DISTANCE		PACE	
HEART RATE		CALORIES		WEATHER	
SHOES		OTHER			

SUNDAY					
RUN TYPE					
ROUTE					
TIME		DISTANCE		PACE	
HEART RATE		CALORIES		WEATHER	
SHOES		OTHER			

NOTES

www.ingramcontent.com/pod-product-compliance
Lightning Source LLC
Chambersburg PA
CBHW070128030426
42335CB00016B/2297